# Chirop

# A Unique Approach to Health.

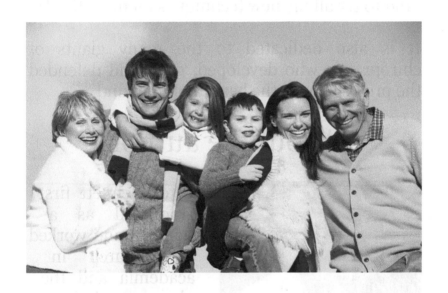

Peter Bennett BSc DC Doctor of Chiropractic

Penrith Family Chiropractic
8 Duke Street, Penrith, CA11 7LY

01768 899 036
www.penrithchiropractic.com

# Dedication

This book is dedicated to my wonderful wife and children who allowed me to pursue my passion (and to try all my new techniques on them first!)

It is also dedicated to the many giants of chiropractic who developed, grew and defended the profession for the benefit of mankind

# About the author

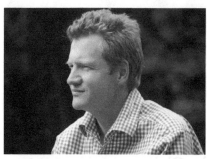 Peter Bennett first graduated as a scientist and worked in research in academia and the pharmaceutical industry. He became a chiropractic patient and was so impressed by the effect that chiropractic had on him that he enrolled in the McTimoney College of Chiropractic in Oxford, graduating in 1998.

After working in Oxfordshire he moved his family

to Cumbria, where he set up Alive Family Wellness in Penrith.

He and his wife and seven children all receive regular chiropractic care. His children have been adjusted since birth to make sure they have an unfair advantage in life.

*"When health is absent Wisdom cannot reveal itself, Art cannot become manifest, Strength cannot be exerted, Wealth is useless and Reason is powerless."*

**Herophilies, 300 B.C.**

3

*Disclaimer*


*The author and publisher have made every effort in composing the material for this book. The information contained in this book is strictly for educational purposes only. If you wish to apply ideas given in this book, you are taking full responsibility for your actions.*

*The author and publisher disclaim any warranties [expressed or implied], merchantability, or suitability with any particular purpose or objective. The author and publisher shall in no event be held liable to any party for any direct, indirect, punitive, special, incidental or other consequential damages arising directly or indirectly from any use of this material, which is provided "as is", and without warranties.*


*Copyrights © 2011 Peter Bennett BSc DC*
*ISBN 978-1-4477-9283-3*

# Table of contents

## Table of Contents

# Introduction

Most people (if they have ever heard of it) think of chiropractic as a "treatment" for back pain, neck pain or headaches.

If that was all there was to it I, and my family, and my clients, would not have received all the benefits we have received from chiropractic care, and I would not have been inspired to leave my comfortable career and train as a chiropractor.

I hope that this report will give you an accurate picture of what chiropractic is, and what it isn't, and what to expect if you decide to come and see us.

Knowledge is power, and I am a passionate believer that your health is your greatest gift. You must have the knowledge to make your own informed decisions about how to look after your health.

If you have further questions or comments after reading this please don't hesitate to contact me.

I hope you enjoy reading this report.

Yours in health


Peter Bennett
Chiropractor

# Chapter 1

# Expectation and health

Doctors of chiropractic are extremely fortunate in that they combine two of the greatest professions in the world: healthcare and teaching. Most people don't think about chiropractors as teachers, but a good one spends almost as much time educating their patients as they do caring for them.

That's because understanding wellness and being healthy can't be separated. To be healthy you have to learn how your body operates and how best to keep yourself well. That includes learning what to expect when you see various healthcare and medical practitioners

Of course many people just walk into a chiropractic office without knowing anything about chiropractic or what it can do for them. Most of them leave happy and healthy but they seldom get the maximum benefit from this incredible healthcare field. Sadly some of them who enter with an inaccurate or unrealistic expectation leave frustrated and unsatisfied.

That is where chiropractic education comes in

Whenever you enter a chiropractic office the chiropractor has an opportunity to educate you about the benefits of regular spinal care. The chiropractor makes sure you understand that the purpose of the care is to examine your spine and see if the vertebrae and nerves are correctly aligned.

If not it could mean you are **subluxated**. Since the nerve fibres pass through the openings in the bones if an opening is restricted the nerve impulses may be altered as well and that will prevent your body from expressing normal function.

We do not diagnose disease or treat your ailments. Our job is not to suppress symptoms or cure your illnesses. However we will give you the most important help possible – a spine free of nervous system interference! Without interference your body will be free to get itself well.

It is quite common in our office for patients to bring in their entire family for chiropractic care. Most patients feel healthier with each visit and they want their spouses, parents and children to get healthier too.

It is very important to us that all of our patients understand that chiropractic isn't going to cure or treat your back pain, neck pain or headaches. Only your own body's inner wisdom can do that. The purpose of chiropractic is to make sure that your inner wisdom can work properly and that your body can heal itself.

I always say to all my patients at the first visit that if your intention is purely to reduce pain then your best option, and your cheapest option, is to take painkillers, but if your intention is to get yourself so healthy that you don't need to show symptoms then you have come to the right place.

By the time people come to us they have usually accumulated many years of repeated damage to their spine. It would be unrealistic to expect all the damage to be repaired in one or two visits, and, because the damage is still there it would be unrealistic to expect pain to go in one or two visits.

# Realistic expectation leads to satisfaction

Luckily most chiropractors do a good job of educating their patients. As a result most patients have a realistic expectation of how they will benefit from the care programme and most are very satisfied with the results

In fact according to a study conducted in 1991 by Gallup eight of every ten chiropractic patients were satisfied with the care received and they felt that most of their expectations were met.

More than 25 million people visit their chiropractor every year making chiropractic the second largest primary healthcare profession in the world. If all these people are to leave their chiropractors office feeling satisfied with the care they received they have to know what to expect in the first place.

If they go in expecting the chiropractor to diagnose and treat their diseases they are bound to be disappointed since that's not what chiropractic is for. On the other hand if they go realising that their health depends on a good nerve supply and the chiropractors job is to eliminate interference to that nerve supply then they will leave feeling confident about their choice.

There are many reasons why patient satisfaction is so important. The vast majority of chiropractors chose their profession because of the strong desire to help others. Many, like myself, were chiropractic patients themselves and experienced first hand the power of the adjustment. Some had been sickly as children or injured as adults and had tried to find medical answers but failed to achieve health until they found chiropractic.

Now these doctors want to offer the same "miracle" to others. Their compassion is their driving force and they know they won't be able to help patients properly unless the patients understand why they are there.

An analogy I like to use is that of the Fire Brigade. The medical profession is like the Fire Brigade. If your house is burning down you need someone to break down the doors, pull out all the people and soak the whole house in water. The chiropractor is more like a handyman who checks the house at regular intervals and make sure everything is working well so that the house is less likely to go on fire. You wouldn't expect a handyman put out a fire and you wouldn't expect a fireman to repair the damage after you put out the fire.

# Chapter 2

# Where it all started

Chiropractic adjustments (although not named as such) have existed for a very long time. Many civilizations have evidence which suggest that this type of treatment was used.

The first recorded spinal manipulation was found in the Chinese Kong Fu writings dated 2650 BC.

A papyrus found in Egypt dating back to 1600 BC describes a treatment for a dislocated jaw.

Various other societies including ancient Babylon, Tibet, Syria, Japan, India and even some North American tribes and South American groups have been using such treatments.

**Hippocrates**, the Father of Medicine (460-370 BC), described manipulative procedures in his monumental work known as the Corpus Hippocrateum. He wrote, ***"Get knowledge of the spine, for this is the requisite for many diseases."***

**Socrates** (469-399 BC) advised, *"If you would seek health, look first to the spine."*

**Herodotus** gained fame curing diseases by correcting spinal abnormalities through therapeutic exercises. Aristotle was critical of Herodotus' tonic-free approach because, *"he made old men young and thus prolonged their lives too greatly."*

**Claudius Galen** (130-202 AD) discovered the relationship between the nervous system of the spine and healing. He wrote, *"Look to the nervous system as the key to maximum health."* He earned the title 'Prince of Physicians' when he relieved the paralysis of the right hand of Eudemas (a prominent Roman scholar) by careful manipulation of his neck.

Physicians who followed Hippocrates relied on nature's healing power to improve health. They focussed on diet, exercise and rest to improve the health of a patient. To quote Hippocrates *"Natural forces within us are the true healers of disease"*

*"The art of healing comes from nature and not from the physician. Therefore,*

*the physician must start from nature with an open mind.* "
-Paracelsus

The ancient Greece and Roman Empires followed Hippocratic studies and methods very closely. Since physical fitness was important in their kingdoms and half of the men were warriors by profession, it was imperative for them to look after themselves with proper diet and exercise. However, as empires fell most of the knowledge they gained from Hippocrates was lost. However, copies and texts continued to circulate with the help of monks and Islamic physicians living in faraway monasteries, seminaries and mosques around the world.

In the western world medical doctors tended to use three basic treatments:- purging with laxatives, bloodletting, and cupping (heated glasses placed on the affected areas to get rid of tumors).

Ordinary people who didn't have access to doctors required the help of folk or lay practitioners. These practitioners included herbalists and bonesetters. Bonesetters in the past could not only fix broken bones of the arms and legs, but also had enough training to perform adjustment of the spine and other joints. They were very popular in the past in European countries for their various practices. One of the most popular bonesetters in the eighteenth century.was actually not a man, but a woman - Sally Map. In Cumbria bonesetters continued to practice very successfully up to the last 20 years.

# The Foundation of Chiropractic

It's not surprising that many people have the wrong idea about what chiropractic is all about. For more than 100 years since it was first developed into a unique healthcare profession in the USA it has been misunderstood and misrepresented.

Partly this was because it was seen as a threat to the supremacy of the medical profession in the USA. Medical doctors of the turn-of-the-century were enjoying a tremendous surge in popularity. When a lay healer named DD Palmer began getting excellent results by adjusting a persons spine by applying force in a specific manner to the vertebrae medical doctors were at first curious and a few even attended classes held by DD and his son BJ.

DD Palmer         BJ Palmer

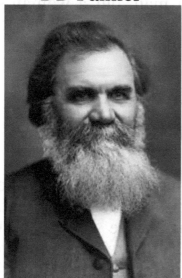 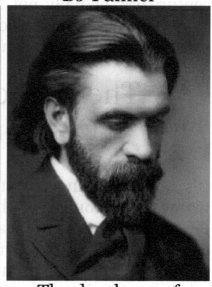

The founder of chiropractic     The developer of chiropractic

But medical doctors didn't like what the Palmers and the new generation of chiropractors were teaching. They were telling students that the best "physicians" in the universe were the patients themselves - that the human body had an **innate intelligence** which kept it constantly striving to achieve better health. If the body was allowed to work without interference, they said, it would reach and maintain its highest possible level of function.

This sounded like some kind of hocus-pocus to the medical doctors who were willing only to believe in scientific evidence they could weigh and measure. They could remove a heart from a corpse and examine it, they could put cells under a microscope and study them, but they couldn't see or even prove the existence of this innate intelligence. The world, they had concluded, was merely an accident of evolution and every movement in it was random.

Physicists today, particularly those studying quantum physics, have taken an 180° turn in scientific thought. Nothing in this universe is truly random. Actually the proof was all around the sceptical doctors but they either couldn't or didn't want to see it. The world definitely was a product of millions of years of evolution but the process was hardly an accident and there was nothing random about the way every creature in the world operated.

Far from being random, the world around us is

very orderly and predictable. Each living creature has an inbuilt knowledge of what it must do to survive and thrive. The circumstances in which it lives might make this impossible to do perfectly, but the knowledge is there.

Take, for example, our own bodies. When we're born we don't have learned knowledge of how to breathe, make our hearts beat, digest our food, or put everything into the right place so we can grow. Luckily our bodies know how to do all these things and the millions of other things which we have to do every second to be alive. Even as we get older, our bodies use their own innate intelligence to function as well as the situation will allow.

When you cut your finger you don't intellectually know how to make a blood clot or how to send extra white blood cells to the area to automatically fight infection. You wouldn't be able to command your body to form a scab to protect the cut area, or to grow new skin cells over the damage. But your body knows how to do these things

Your body also knows how to adapt when you're exposed to germs and viruses, eat a spoiled piece of food or strain your back lifting a heavy object. Whether it will be able to react the way it should depends on the state of your physical body

Because of genetic and environmental factors, the bodies we are born with are not always in perfect condition. In addition, the way we treat our bodies, our diet, lifestyle and emotional and mental attitudes have tremendous effects on our physical condition. If the body is limited by either inherent or acquired weaknesses innate intelligence alone will not be able to achieve perfect health. But it will always keep trying and working in that direction.

Perhaps the most important component, often overlooked even by popular alternative doctors is **spinal nerve interference**, and this is where chiropractic comes in.

The body's nervous system is an incredibly complex communication network which links the brain to all parts of the body, chemically influencing even the smallest cells. There are miles of nerve fibres running throughout our bodies. No one has been able to count the number of nerve cells in the human body but it is estimated that there are at least 10 to

12,000,000,000 of them, possibly many, many more.

Over this nerve network the brain receives constantly updated information from the cells, organs and tissues and instantaneously relays instructions back. The whole process is so fast that scientists have only recently begun to measure the speed of impulses and no one has come up with a definitive speed. But you can get an idea of the incredible speed by remembering what happened last time you grabbed hold of the handle of a hot pot on the stove

Before you even realised what had happened, you jerked your hand away - and immediately a blister started forming as a protective response to the injury. You hardly had a chance to cry out in pain, but the cells in your finger had already transmitted the information about the injury to your brain which responded by instructing the cells to react in a specific way determined by your innate intelligence.

That's exactly what happens with every other cell in your body, all the time. You don't have to burn yourself to trigger the communication system. The flow of information to and from your body is a constant background function which keeps your body as healthy as it can be given its specific physical limitations.

But what if something interferes with the communication system? What if there is "line noise" as they call it in telephone circuits? What if the messages to and from the brain become even the slightest bit garbled?

The results can range from a slightly less than perfect response of a particular tissue cell, to a steadily worsening malfunction of a vital organ or life-support system. Either way, your body is not going to be able to do what its innate intelligence knows it has to do to keep up optimal health.

The spine is made up of 24 small bones called vertebrae: seven in the neck (**cervical**); 12 in the mid-back (**thoracic**) and five in the lower back (**lumbar**). Most of these vertebrae are shaped somewhat like doughnuts with a hole in the middle. The spinal-cord fits into, and is protected by, these ring shaped bones. Two additional vertebrae at the bottom of the spine, the **sacrum** and the **coccyx**, complete what is called the **spinal column**.

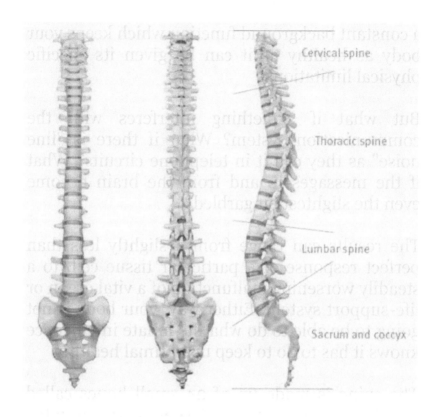

Cervical spine

Thoracic spine

Lumbar spine

Sacrum and coccyx

Naturally, nerve endings have to be able to branch out throughout the whole body, so the spinal column isn't merely a solid bone casing. Instead it is a marvel of engineering design.

The bones stack together in a precise way which allows a "canal" between them, aptly called the **"neural canal"**. It is through this small canal that the primary nerve bundles branch off the spinal cord and make their way to all parts of the body.

If we didn't have to bend, those bones could have been locked into place. But the spine has to be flexible so its design incorporates a thick fibrous cushion of cartilage, called an **intervertebral disk**, which acts as a shock absorber, in the joint between each pair of vertebrae. This allows us to bend, turn, flex or move with relative freedom

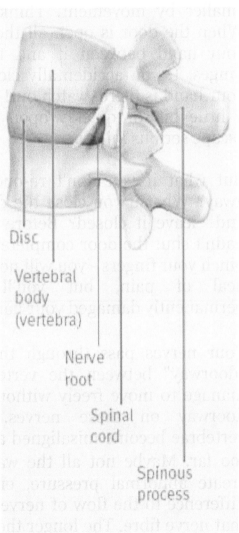

Disc

Vertebral body (vertebra)

Nerve root

Spinal cord

Spinous process

Unfortunately this need for flexibility means that the size of the canals can be made larger or smaller by movement. Think of it as a door. When the door is open all the way you can put your hand between it and the wall near the hinges. If you accidentally close the door when your hand is there, watch out! If you close it only a little bit, or quickly open it again you may escape serious injury.

But what if you don't re-open the door right away? What if you close the door on your hand and leave it closed? Before long, even if you hadn't shut the door completely - just enough to pinch your fingers - you will not only be in a great deal of pain, but you'll probably have permanently damaged your hand.

Your nerves pass through the opening in the "doorway" between the vertebrae. Usually we manage to move freely without ever closing the doorway on these nerves. But sometimes vertebrae become misaligned and the door shuts too far. Maybe not all the way, just enough to create abnormal pressure, enough to make a difference to the flow of nerve impulses through that nerve fibre. The longer the door is left partly closed the worst the damage will be.

When vertebrae become stuck in an abnormal position it's called a **vertebral subluxation**. To be more precise the subluxation is not merely the presence of the misaligned bone it also involves the presence of a **"neurological insult"** to use the technical term. In other words the misalignment is causing a 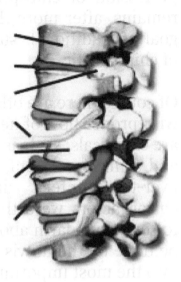 change in the flow of normal impulses. The nerve "short-circuits" and is being disrupted in some way because of the misaligned bones.

The effects of vertebral subluxation on health have been well-documented in the millions of case studies recorded by practising chiropractors. It is the chiropractor's job to determine whether there are any subluxations and to introduce the precise amount of force, called an **adjustment**, to gently but firmly unlock the vertebrae and allow them to return to the proper alignment.

This is the single purpose for which the profession of chiropractic was founded, and it remains, after more than a century, the primary goal of traditional, subluxation centred, doctors of chiropractic.

Of course there are other things that can interfere with proper flow of nerve impulses. Among these are chemicals, such as those found in certain food and drinks, pollutants and even prescription and over-the-counter drugs. In fact early chiropractors were the first **"body ecologists"** to sound an alarm about the damage which could be done by the unwise use of chemicals dumped into the most important stream in the world - the human bloodstream.

They taught that people can't expect to take a magic pill to improve the function of the body. DD Palmer expressed this with the phrase **"above down, inside out".** He meant that true health comes from within - not from without.

Obviously this didn't sit well with the evolving medical establishment, which was coming to rely more and more heavily on drugs and surgery to "treat" patients. Doctors began focusing all their attention on "scientific breakthroughs" - from antibiotics to iron lungs.

For these upstart chiropractors to tell patients they had the power within themselves to heal and become healthy was an outrage. Patients needed medical doctors to give them drugs, more hospitals to operate on their organs, deliver their babies and scientifically treat their diseases. Chiropractors were "quacks" to be avoided at all cost.

Under all this pressure the very small number of chiropractors in the USA at the start of the twentieth century were struggling to keep going. Then something happened that raised the profile of chiropractic and boosted its growth – the 1918 Spanish Flu pandemic. It has been estimated that 20 million people died throughout the world, including about 500,000 Americans. It was chiropractic's success in caring for flu victims that led to the profession's acceptance in many states of the USA.

Researchers reported that in Davenport, Iowa, out of the 93,590 patients treated by medical doctors, there were 6,116 deaths -- a loss of one patient out of every 15.

Chiropractors at the Palmer School of Chiropractic adjusted 1,635 cases, with only one death.

Outside Davenport, chiropractors in Iowa cared for 4,735 cases with only six deaths -- one out of 866.

During the same epidemic, in Oklahoma, out of 3,490 flu patients under chiropractic care, there were only seven deaths. Furthermore, chiropractors were called in 233 cases given up as lost after medical treatment, and reportedly saved all but 25.

By the middle of the 20th century the medical profession was working hard to bring everyone into the medical model of sickness and disease care. Today, the medical, hospital and drug industries pump billions of pounds into advertising and marketing in order to keep the public convinced that the **allopathic** (treatment of symptoms from the outside) medical model is the only viable system.

Despite this chiropractic has grown to be the second largest healthcare profession in the world with millions of adjustments delivered every day.

# Chapter 3

# Why people are confused

**The definition of chiropractic is simple: a health care system dedicated to the detection and correction of vertebral subluxation to eliminate spinal nerve interference. It is also drug-free, non-invasive and works with your body's own innate striving for health. That's it – pure, simple and powerful.**

So why do people get confused about what chiropractic is?

There are a number of reasons

# Well meaning patients cause confusion.

First there are all those testimonials from satisfied patients. Of course chiropractors love to hear from patients who are feeling healthier and happier because of regular chiropractic care. But, as we mentioned before, some patients forget the most important important part of the story - that correcting vertebral subluxation allows the intelligence that made the body to heal the body. In their enthusiasm they give credit to the chiropractor for their "cures".

When a patient tells a friend that her child's ear infections were "cured" by chiropractic the friend is bound to get the impression that the chiropractor diagnosed the child's condition and specifically treated it. The same thing goes when a patient tells a co-worker that his migraines disappeared after only a few adjustments. The co-worker will go home thinking chiropractic is a treatment for headaches.

When the friend and the co-worker go to see the chiropractor themselves, they going to be expecting their chiropractor to diagnose their illnesses and treat them. When they're told that the purpose of chiropractic is to determine whether they have subluxations in their spine and correct them, they are bound to be confused.

One way to avoid this confusion is for us to make sure that patients have proper educational material- hence this report.

For their part patients have to play an active role in their own healthcare and take time to learn about and understand chiropractic.

This isn't easy because for decades we've been made to be spectators when it comes to health. We sit back and put our health into the hands of the experts. Studies have shown that the vast majority of patients who go to a medical doctor never ask a single question about the doctor's diagnosis or treatment plan. They never ask about the drugs they are given, not even about potential side-effects they may experience. Most are too intimidated to demand a second opinion even in the case of the diagnosis of serious illness. This is as much a problem for the medical doctor as it is the patient. If there is no dialogue the doctor can miss out on important information.

Your health is too important not to ask questions about your care, your chiropractic care or your medical care. If you don't take the time to understand what they can do for you and how they are going to do it you're not going to get as much out of it as those people who are well informed, and you risk the dissatisfaction that comes with misunderstanding.

# Deliberately misleading the public

As we noted in the previous chapter, medical doctors were at first curious about this new health care field. They quickly became afraid of it. If people adopted it as their primary approach to health there would be less need for medical doctors and their drugs, surgery and therapies.

During the early years of chiropractic in the USA there was no such thing as a chiropractic licence. Medical doctors who had to pass tests to get their licenses to practice were angry about losing patients to people who were in their eyes, "laymen". As healthcare was private this meant loss of income for them. To stop this exodus of patients, medical doctors tried put their chiropractic competitors out of business by accusing them of practising medicine without a licence.

Medical doctors would often hire people to go to a chiropractor pretending to be a patient. The chiropractor would do their work, and would then be reported for practising medicine without a licence. Most of the early chiropractors spent some time in prison, and some were in and out of prison so often that they set up busy practices within the prisons, thus giving great benefit to the prisoners and staff!

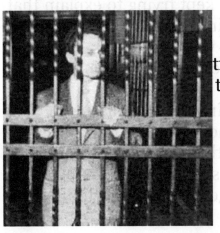
Dr Herbert Ross Reaver went to jail 13 times in 11 years rather than admit to the false charge that he was practising medicine without a licence

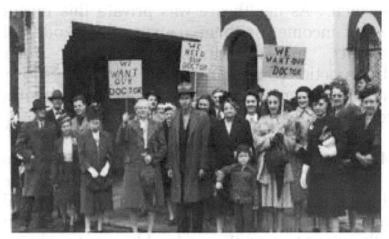

Dr Reaver's patients protesting over his tenth
imprisonment

Throughout it all chiropractors kept practising
chiropractic and kept attracting new patients as
the word spread. They kept trying to explain that
they were not diagnosing and treating conditions
and diseases, as that was medicine's job. They
were finding and correcting subluxations.

Despite the continuing harassment of
chiropractors chiropractic kept growing because
people kept referring their friends and family to
the chiropractor because they were so happy with
the results they were getting. This led to the next
problem.

# Credited with cures.

Incredible "success" stories started circulating from satisfied patients. "It cured my arthritis" one would say. Another would tell a story about a baby who had colic and had been taking medication for months – but was "cured" by a few chiropractic adjustments. Others claimed it stopped their migraines or cleared up their allergies.

Chiropractors found it necessary to keep emphasising that these miraculous "cures" were the direct result of unleashing the patient's own natural healing power from within. The chiropractors refused to claim the credit for any improvement in the patient's health, knowing that the patient was healing themselves.

Eventually chiropractic was established as a separate profession with its own education and licensing and chiropractors were allowed to legally open practices. The number of patients attending chiropractors continued to grow and so did the claims of "cures" from patients.

# Taking it to court

The American Medical Association (AMA) spent millions of dollars in an attempt to destroy chiropractic. For years the AMA released a barrage of misinformation to the public and to its own members. It forbade its members from associating with, or referring patients to chiropractors. Having anything to do with chiropractors was considered unethical and unprofessional.

Finally in 1976 a group of chiropractors decided to fight back. They spent years gathering evidence to prove their contention that the medical community has engaged in the in a deliberate attempt to eliminate competition by maligning chiropractic.

The AMA claimed it was acting in the best interests of patients since chiropractic was not only ineffective but dangerous. However the chiropractors brought in their own evidence which showed chiropractic was safe and effective.

The chiropractors won and the AMA and its co-defendants were found guilty of conspiracy to create a medical monopoly. On August 27, 1987 US district Court Judge Susan Getzendanner issued her opinion that as far back as 1963 the AMA had been working aggressively both "overtly and covertly" to eliminate the profession of chiropractic. She issued a permanent court injunction against the AMA to prevent such behaviour in future.

However there is still a great deal of misinformation about chiropractic in the media. Sometimes articles come out about the dangers of **spinal manipulation**, implying that chiropractic is dangerous. However in these cases the spinal manipulation was often performed by doctors, physiotherapists or other health professionals, not by chiropractors.

It is important to realise the difference between spinal manipulation and adjustment. Spinal manipulation is an "outside-in" procedure – it involves the therapist making the patient's spine go where the therapist thinks it should go. This can be painful (and sometimes dangerous) if the patient's spine disagrees with the therapist!

Adjustment is an "inside-out" procedure – the chiropractor finds out where the patient's innate intelligence is trying to put the spine and nudge it in the required direction. Because the spine is not being forced it is a safer approach.

In recent years, the campaign against chiropractic has changed. The campaigners have realised that they can't destroy chiropractic – but they are still hoping to limit it.

Chiropractic today is often depicted as a last resort "treatment" for low back pain in adults – a sort of alternative physiotherapy.

Despite all this, more than 25 million people visit their chiropractors each year on every continent, most of them having heard of chiropractic by word of mouth.

Hundreds of millions of adjustments are performed every year and chiropratic continues to be safe and effective. I'm proud that my professional  insurance costs less than my car insurance – and I'm a safe driver!

But the continued assault on chiropractic over the decades has had a lasting effect on the public's perception of chiropractic and of health in general. Most have never come across the idea that their own bodies have an innate ability to heal.

# Confusion amongst chiropractors themselves.

As chiropractic has been under attack, and as the education to become a chiropractor has become more intense and more involved, some chiropractic colleges have included more and more medical education and procedures. Sometimes the graduates of these colleges have forgotten that the medical content of their course is designed to enable chiropractors to recognise when the patient needs to see a medical practitioner, not to enable the chiropractor to become more medical.

In our practice we try to keep this as clear as possible. This is why I don't use my Dr title, I don't wear a white coat, and I don't use stethoscopes or any medical equipment. My patients see me for chiropractic issues, and their medical doctor for medical issues.

# Chapter 4

## The chiropractic examination for vertebral subluxation

As you have read, the focus of our practice is to improve your health by detecting and correcting vertebral subluxations (interference to your nerves).

Therefore our examinations are aimed very specifically at this focus.

The initial questionnaire is designed to get as much information as possible to help us decide whether you should come to us, or whether you should see your GP in the first instance.

The examinations are designed to find the effect of subluxation on your body.

## Physical examination

This will include the following tests

# Range of motion.

One of the effects of the vertical subluxation is to impair voluntary movement (called **"dyskinesia"**). In patients this usually means difficulty turning their head or body from side to side or front to back. Often patients will be able to turn to the left a lot further than they can to the right or vice versa. This impaired range of motion can be tested and measured very accurately.

# Postural checks

The way you hold your body can be a good indication of the proper alignment of the spine. We will visually check various reference points and note the tilt and balance of each. A patient who stands with one shoulder higher than the other, for example, might have a severe vertebral subluxation which could cause serious health damage.

# Leg length check

If your body is compensating for subluxations in your spine you will twist yourself and you will end up with one leg longer than the other. Most people have one leg longer than the other, but this is because most people are subluxated. People under our care always have even leg length, (unless they have had leg surgery or a bad fracture)

# Palpation

After years of chiropractic college training and clinical practice chiropractors learn to "feel" for subluxations in the spine with the tips of the fingers. Most are remarkably accurate with this type of examination and can also become aware of any tenderness, soreness or discomfort experienced by the patient as a result of having vertical subluxations.

# Instrumentation

In the last 10 years chiropractic examinations

have become much more sophisticated

We perform **surface electromyography (sEMG)** to measure the electrical energy expended by the body. This is important since another key component of vertebral subluxation is what is known as **"dysponesis"** or abnormal involuntary muscle activity.

In these scans white is normal, green is mild disruption, blue is moderate and red is severe disruption. Black is very severe disruption.

Below is an example of the results of a sEMG scan. This was an 8 year old with cerebral palsy. He was using a walking frame and had both legs in splints. We can't reproduce the colours here so look at the length of the bars – the longer the bar is the more disruption there is to nerve function.

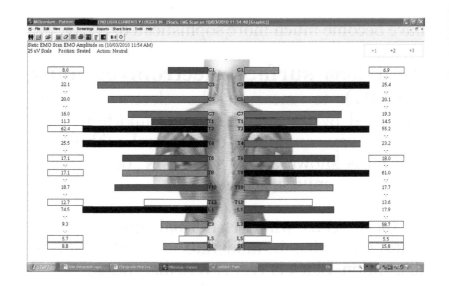

## This is the same child after 14 visits.

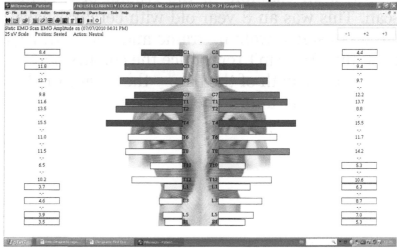

As you can see the nervous system is more

balanced and under less stress. He still had the cerebral palsy but we had helped to reduce the effects of the cerebral palsy on his nervous system. He was now walking without the frame and playing football with his dad in the garden.

**Surface thermography** measures skin temperature to spot abnormalities in the autonomic nervous system (which automatically controls the behaviour of the cells and organs) This is the surface thermography scan of a lady in her 50s before starting care.

As before, white is normal, green is mild disruption, blue is moderate and red is severe disruption. In this example you can see the first scan has coloured bars, showing disruption, and the second scan does not.

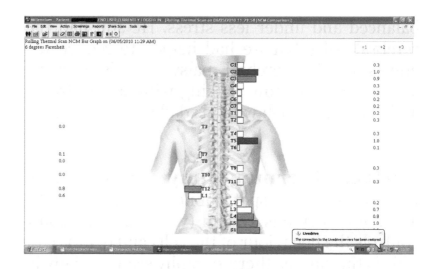

This is the same lady after 12 adjustments.

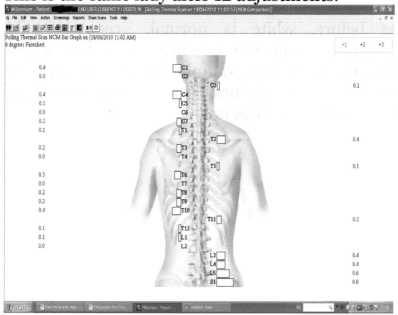

It is important to stress again that none of these tests are designed to diagnose medical conditions. We will be alert for signs that the patient should see a medical doctor, but we do not do medical diagnosis.

We explain what we have found, and what we can do about it. You then decide whether to carry on with care.

# Chapter 5

# Frequently asked questions

## Do I have to get undressed?

In our office the only time you need to remove any clothes is for the scan. This is because we take the readings from the skin next to your spine. I would leave the room while you remove only your shirt or blouse (ladies leave their bra on) and put on a hospital gown open at the back. After the scan I leave the room again while you get dressed. You remain fully clothed at all other times.

## Will you "crack my bones"?

Many of my patients have this concern at their first visit, probably because of the confusion over spinal manipulation as opposed to spinal adjustment. (see page 39). Because I'm working with your body rather than forcing it to do things

I am very gentle. In fact the usual response after the first adjustment is "Is that all you need to do?"

## Why do I have to be adjusted so frequently?

Everyone is unique so everyone will have a different care plan set out for them. There are a number of reasons why people need different care

1. As you have accumulated problems with the nervous system and the spine over years there'll be layers of scar tissue. The scar tissue and tissue damage makes the spine unstable and it tends to revert back to what it is used to. Until the tissues have regrown in the correct place the adjustments have to be frequently repeated to keep the nerves clear.

2. As you have adapted to your spinal problems over the years you would have developed postural habits - for example holding your head to one side or hitching your pelvis up on one side. Your central nervous system has recorded these postural habits and you have a tendency to revert

back to what you think is normal. Again repeated adjustments retrain the postural habits.

3. Many of the stresses that caused the subluxations in the first place are still ongoing - physical and emotional and chemical. Over time we try to eliminate the stresses but not all of them can be eliminated. Initially we are trying to remove subluxations faster than you can put them back in again.

# Do I have to follow the schedule of visits that my chiropractor has recommended?

You don't have to do anything you don't want to! The whole approach of chiropractic is to make you the centre of all that we do – you are in control. This also means that you are responsible for your healthcare. Your chiropractor will tell you what, in his opinion is the minimal amount of care that you will need to reach your health objectives. If you decide you don't want that level of health just discuss this with your chiropractor. However, don't expect to get Rolls Royce health if you are only paying for Ford Cortina health!

# What reactions I likely to get?

## Feeling worse before you get better

Once your innate intelligence is able to start working on the damage to your body your body's response is to break down scar tissue and replace it. The process by which this is done is inflammation. Sometimes inflammation causes pain and you can feel worse before you get better. Sometimes it takes several weeks of care before the nervous system is clear enough for your innate intelligence to break down scar tissue. In these cases patients will initially feel better for a few weeks and then have a few days of pain while the inflammation process proceeds.

# Body chemistry changes

As the innate intelligence is dealing with the new information flowing through the nervous system the activity of all the cells in the body can be corrected. This involves changes to body chemistry which can lead to reactions such as emotional changes, heavy sleep or light sleep and changes in the need for medication such as blood pressure medication. The body will always settle itself quickly to as near normal as it can manage so all of these reactions settle down. In some cases the need for medication use will be reduced. Changes in medication should be discussed with your medical doctor.

## Retracing of old trauma

I have seen cases where the patient has experienced severe physical or emotional trauma at some point in the past. In some cases this trauma has been recorded in the body and will come out and be processed under chiropractic care. Again this is a temporary effect.

The body can change in many ways. Always ask your chiropractor about any symptoms or reactions that you are concerned about.

# What is that popping noise I sometimes hear during an adjustment?

If a joint has been under stress and been twisted or compressed there will sometimes be a "pop" or "crack" when it releases. As the joint space is opened up the reduction in pressure in the joint fluid causes a gas bubble to form. When the joint settles into it's new postion the bubble pops – making the noise. No damage is being caused.

# Why does have my chiropractor seem to do less work on me in some visits than in others?

The aim of the visit is make sure that any subluxations in your nervous system are resolved. Ideally we will have got the timing of your appointments about right so you won't have accumulated many subluxations and there won't be a lot to adjust. On other visits there may be a lot of adjustments because you have been under stress. Remember that we will check everything in your nervous system at every visit.

# Why are the appointments short?

Remember that the aim of the visit is make sure that any subluxations in your nervous system are resolved. The techniques we use have been developed over the last 100+ years to quickly identify the issues that your body wants to deal with. When the primary subluxation is dealt with the secondary subluxations will often be resolved at the same time. The core part of each visit will often take about a minute. We allow time for double checking and for you to ask questions and so on, but even so we have found about five minutes is enough.

The only thing you can't get more of is time. We find that people usually prefer short appointments. It allows them to fit the appointments into their busy lives. It also allows us to be very flexible in moving appointments about to suit you.

However we don't want you to feel rushed. If you feel you need more time with us please ask. We can easily do this and there is no extra charge.

# What sort of issues have been helped by chiropractic?

Remember that the purpose of chiropractic is not to treat symptoms but to clear the nervous system and allow innate intelligence to function. This has resulted in many changes to people's health.

The following is a sampling of published research over the last twenty years, just to give you an impression of the possible effects of letting the innate intelligence work properly.

# Chapter 6

# A selection of published research

## Patient satisfaction

**Patient Satisfaction With Chiropractic Physicians in an Independent Physicians' Association**
**J Manipulative Physiol Ther 2001 (Nov); 24 (9): 556–559**

Various aspects of chiropractic care were given a rating of "excellent" by the following percentage of respondents: Length of time to get an appointment (84.9%); convenience of the office (57.7%); access to the office by telephone (77.3%); length of wait at the office (75.7%); time spent with the provider (74.3%); explanation of what was done during the visit (72.8%); technical skills of the chiropractor (83.3%); and the personal manner of the chiropractor (92.4%). The visit overall was rated as excellent by 83.3% of responders, and 95.3% stated they would definitely recommend the provider to others

## The Gallup Study

In 1991 the Gallup Organization performed a nationwide demographic study to determine the attitudes, opinions, and behaviors of both users and nonusers of chiropractic services.

Overall, 90% felt that chiropractic health care was effective: more than 80% were satisfied with the treatment they received; nearly 75% felt that most of their expectations were met during the last visit or series of visits; 68% said they would likely see a doctor of chiropractic again for treatment of a similar condition, and 50% would likely be willing to see a doctor of chiropractic for some other problem chiropractors treat. Nearly 80% of the chiropractic users felt that the cost of chiropractic treatment was reasonable.

Demographic Characteristics of Users of

Chiropractic Services. The Gallup
Organization, Princeton, New Jersey – 1991

According to this 1994 Harris Poll, patients
were more satisfied with chiropractic care
than care from medical doctors and other
health care professionals.

Those who sought care from a chiropractor
were more likely to be very satisfied with
their care than those who visited any other
practitioner. (Choices were between
Chiropractic Doctors, Medical Doctors,
Physical Therapists, or Osteopathic
Doctors) Of those who have seen both types
of practitioner, the majority were more
likely to be satisfied with the care of the
chiropractor than with that of the medical
doctor.

1994 Harris Poll

Patient Evaluations of Care from
Family Physicians and Chiropractors

Findings from this study indicate that patients under chiropractic care had 3 times the satisfaction rate as did patients under the care of Family Physicians. In addition, the patient's perception of the doctor's confidence in diagnosing and treating low back pain was almost 3 times higher in patients receiving chiropractic care compared with those receiving care from family physicians.

**Patient Evaluations of Care from Family Physicians and Chiropractors**
Western Journal of Medicine 1989 (Mar); 150 (3): 351–355

# Safety of chiropractic care

A Risk Assessment of Cervical Manipulation vs. NSAIDs for the Treatment of Neck Pain Dabbs V, Lauretti WJ  J Manipulative Physiol Ther 1995 (Oct);  18 (8):  530–536

CONCLUSION:  The best evidence indicates that cervical manipulation for neck pain is much safer than the use of NSAIDs, by as much as a factor of several hundred times. There is no evidence that indicates NSAID use is any more effective than

# Costs and outcomes of chiropractic care

**Comparative Analysis of Individuals With and Without Chiropractic Coverage: Patient Characteristics, Utilization, and Costs**
**Archives of Internal Medicine 2004 (Oct 11);   164 (18):   1985–1892**

A 4-year retrospective claims data analysis comparing more than 700,000 health plan members within a managed care environment found that **members had lower annual total health care expenditures, utilized x-rays and MRIs less, had less back surgeries**, and for patients with chiropractic coverage, compared with those without coverage, **also had lower average back pain episode-related costs ($289 vs $399)**.

**The authors concluded:** "**Access to managed chiropractic care may reduce overall health care expenditures through several effects, including** (1) positive risk selection; **(2) substitution of chiropractic for traditional medical care, particularly for spine conditions**; (3) more conservative, less invasive treatment profiles; and (4) lower health service costs associated with managed chiropractic care."

## Self-reported Nonmusculoskeletal Responses to Chiropractic Intervention: A Multination Survey
**J Manipulative Physiol Ther 2005 (Jun); 28 (5): 294–302**
Positive reactions were reported by 2% to 10% of all patients and by 3% to 27% of those who reported to have such problems. Most common were improved breathing (27%), digestion (26%), and circulation (21%).

# Chiropractic and DNA repair

Campbell CJ, Kent C, Banne A, Amiri A, Pero RW: "Surrogate indication of DNA repair in serum after long term chiropractic intervention a retrospective study." *Journal of Vertebral*

*Subluxation Research* [February 18, 2005, pp 15]. http://www.jvsr.com

Kent C: "Assessment of DNA repair, autonomic tone, and paraspinal muscle tone in a population of long term chiropractic patients: a pilot study." Conference Abstracts. International Research and Philosophy Symposium. Sherman College of Straight Chiropractic. Spartanburg, SC. October 910, 2004. http://www.sherman.edu/edu/research/pdf/IRAPS _abstracts_2004.pdf

# Chapter 7

# Some of our clients' stories

**Gary**, a professional musician, came in for his fourth visit. To quote him "I'm really delighted with the way my back pain has cleared up so quickly. I played a gig on Saturday and had no back pain for the first time in many months"

Gary knows that I haven't cured him - I have cleared the interference from his nerves and he is in the process of healing himself.

The quality of his life has improved because he can now do what he loves - playing in a band - without anything affecting his focus and concentration and taking away the joy.

**George**. "I've been telling everybody that this is the first time in 20 odd years that I haven't been waking up every single morning with nagging pain in my low back. Now I am waking with no pain and better rested."

## Another reason I love what I do

A 10 month old little girl was brought to see me in May 2010. She had had a very traumatic birth. She had to go immediately into resuscitation for 24 minutes. Then 2 hours after delivery she suffered a series of seizures that continued for 10 days. Her parents were told that she was brain damaged and would never see, hear or respond and would never walk.

She was taken to see a fellow chiropractor in February 2010 and transferred to me in May.

She and her family were in our reception in March 2011. When I walked in she saw me and smiled! She can now respond to her family and giggles and laughs at her brothers' antics. When they left she smiled and waved to us.


A farmer came in with knee pain which hadn't eased in over a month.

I examined him, carried out a nerve function scan, and talked him through the results.

I explained that I don't "treat" knee pain - I just

correct subluxations so that his innate intelligence would do its' work.

He looked at me as if I was mad, but consented to being adjusted.

As he got off the bench and stood up a big grin spread over his face - "The pain's all gone - is that supposed to happen?"

On his third visit he said "You know you were talking about them nerve thingies. Well since my first visit I can think straighter, and I'm not feeling like my food is coming back up my throat when I go to bed at night. Is that anything to do with getting my nerves working properly?"


A lady in her 60s had been suffering from at least two migraines per month for the last 15 years.

The scan of her motor nerves and autonomic nerves performed at her first visit in February 2010 severe disruption in her upper neck.

She received chiropractic care twice a week for the first 4 weeks, once a week for the next 4 weeks, then once a fortnight for 4 months. She is now checked once a month.

When the scans were repeated in August

2010 there was still some disruption but it was greatly reduced.

This lady has had <u>no migraines since April 2010</u>

# Summary

The sole purpose of chiropractic care is to make sure that your body is able to communicate fully with your brain so that every part of your body works the way it is supposed to.

That is it – the sum total

The reason I get adjusted regularly and I adjust my family regularly is the same reason we eat well, and the same reason we exercise, and the same reason we take care about how we think and what we think about.

My personal belief is that you can't be fully alive and healthy without a fully functioning nervous system, and you can't have that unless you get adjusted and take care of your body.

That is my personal belief. I don't expect it to be anyone else's belief. My responsibility as a chiropractor is to take care of your health in the best way I can, to the level you want to be cared for.

Whether you want relief of your symptoms or the

fullest health possible I will honour your wishes.
Chiropractic is, and always has been, about you.

Yours in health

Peter

#0146 - 200318 - C0 - 210/148/4 - PB - DID2153475